Simulation Simplified

STUDENT LAB MANUAL FOR CRITICAL CARE NURSING

Sandra Goldsworthy, RN, MSc, CNCC, CMSN
Coordinator Critical Care e-Learning Program
Durham College
Assistant Professor
Collaborative BScN Program
Durham College/University of Ontario
 Institute of Technology

Leslie Graham, RN, MN, CNCC
Professor, Nursing
BScN Collaborative Nursing Program
Critical Care e-Learning Certificate Program
Durham College

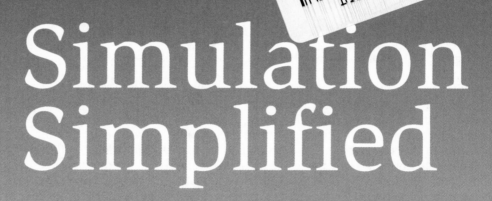
Wolters Kluwer | Lippincott Williams & Wilkins
Health
Philadelphia • Baltimore • New York • London
Buenos Aires • Hong Kong • Sydney • Tokyo

Senior Acquisitions Editor: Elizabeth Nieginski
Digital Acquisitions Editor: John Jordan
Product Manager: Eric Van Osten
Design Coordinator: Joan Wendt
Illustration Coordinator: Brett MacNaughton
Manufacturing Coordinator: Karin Duffield
Prepress Vendor: Aptara, Inc.

9 8 7 6 5 4 3 2 1

Printed in the United States of America

ISBN: 978-1-4511-4469-7

Care has been taken to confirm the accuracy of the information presented and to describe generally accepted practices. However, the authors, editors, and publisher are not responsible for errors or omissions or for any consequences from application of the information in this book and make no warranty, expressed or implied, with respect to the currency, completeness, or accuracy of the contents of the publication. Application of this information in a particular situation remains the professional responsibility of the practitioner; the clinical treatments described and recommended may not be considered absolute and universal recommendations.

The authors, editors, and publisher have exerted every effort to ensure that drug selection and dosage set forth in this text are in accordance with the current recommendations and practice at the time of publication. However, in view of ongoing research, changes in government regulations, and the constant flow of information relating to drug therapy and drug reactions, the reader is urged to check the package insert for each drug for any change in indications and dosage and for added warnings and precautions. This is particularly important when the recommended agent is a new or infrequently employed drug.

Some drugs and medical devices presented in this publication have Food and Drug Administration (FDA) clearance for limited use in restricted research settings. It is the responsibility of the health care provider to ascertain the FDA status of each drug or device planned for use in his or her clinical practice.

LWW.com

To my wonderful husband and children, for without their constant support this project would not have been possible

To all of the critical care nursing students I have had the privilege of mentoring over the years

Sandra Goldsworthy

To my family for their ongoing love and support, always

To my nursing mentors who give so willingly

Leslie Graham

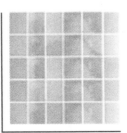

Video Reviewers

Annette Bourgault, PhD(c), MSc, RN, CNCC(C), CNL
Clinical Nurse Leader Program Director, Dept. of Physiological and
  Technological Nursing
Georgia Health Sciences University
Augusta, Georgia, USA

Janet Piper, RegN, MScN, CCRN(c)
Health Sciences Lab Specialist, Simulation Laboratory
Sault College of Applied Arts and Technology
Sault Ste. Marie, ON, Canada

Leland J. Rockstraw, PhD, RN
Associate Clinical Professor of Nursing & Assistant Dean, Simulation,
  Clinical & Technology Learning Operations
Drexel University - College of Nursing & Health Professions
Philadelphia, Pennsylvania, USA

Dr. Colin Torrance RN, DipLScN, BSc(Hon), PhD
Professor in Health Professional Education/Head of Simulation
University of Glamorgan, Glyntaff Campus
Pontypridd, UK

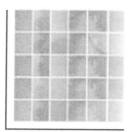

Preface

Welcome to *Simulation Simplified*! This text has been designed for nurses in critical care programs or in undergraduate nursing programs. This resource will also be very helpful to critical care nurses who desire to update their skills by learning through hands-on comprehensive critical care simulation cases. The goal of this book is to promote excellence in simulation education and critical care nursing practice.

The lessons learned from this text and accompanying electronic resources will help take the mystery, guess work, and difficulty out of the components of transitioning into the critical care workplace. You will learn how to care for critically ill patients in a variety of circumstances. The simulation cases were created to imitate the critical care practice setting through a realistic portrayal of patient cases. In addition, you will learn how to reflect on your learning by participating in high quality debriefing/reflective thinking sessions after the simulation has been implemented. This text provides a practical approach to learning the essential competencies required to care for a critically ill patient.

An Overview of *Simulation Simplified*:
Simulation Simplified consists of an instructor text, a student handbook, and accompanying electronic resources. The student handbook is composed of 10 chapters. Each chapter is related to a specific topic of patient care. In addition, you will find many helpful step-by-step guides to assist you in performing such skills as: arterial blood gas analysis, arrhythmia interpretation, and a guide to participating in family conferences. Each chapter is based on a specific topic (ie, Myocardial Infarction, Hypovolemic Shock) and includes practice pre-test and post-test questions as well as suggested readings to prepare for the simulation lab. Every case has an accompanying video vignette that you can view of the case before attending the simulation lab to participate in the case.

Features
- Learning Objectives
- Each chapter begins with a list of learning objectives that will assist the reader to focus his or her reading.

References
A list of current references cited in the chapter is given at the end of each chapter.

Appendices

The appendices include many helpful guides for you to use both within the simulation lab and in the critical care practice area. Included are the following:

- Systematic Approach to Arrhythmia Interpretation
- Systematic Approach to 12 lead ECG Interpretation
- Vasoactive Drip Calculation Formulas
- Arterial Blood Gas Interpretation
- Pulmonary Artery Waveforms Guide
- Critical Care Pharmacology Table
- Abnormal Lab Values and Assessment Table
- Hemodynamic Algorithm
- Family Conference Protocol

Electronic Resources

Electronic instructor resources for *Simulation Simplified* include the following:

- Ten complete video vignette critical care simulation cases. These cases are designed to accompany the 10 cases outlined in the instructor text and the accompanying student handbook.
- Suggested pre-reading for all 10 cases.
- ThePoint. (http://thepoint.lww.com) It is a web-based course and content management system that provides every resource, instructors' and students' need in one easy-to-use site. Advanced technology and superior content combine at thePoint to allow instructors to design and deliver online and offline courses. Students can visit thePoint to access supplemental multimedia resources and enhance their learning experience.
- Access to regularly updated information used for reference in hospital settings: Lippincott's Nursing Advisor and Lippincott's Nursing Procedures and Skills. See the Simulation Simplified access card for more details.

It is with great pleasure we introduce these resources—the instructor textbook, the student handbook, and the online package—to you. One of our primary goals in creating these resources has been to promote excellence in critical care nursing simulation practice so that nurses can enhance their skills in a safe environment and ultimately increase the levels of high quality, safe patient care. It is our intent that these resources will provide critical care educators and nurses, both in the academic and practice setting, with practical strategies for application in order to deliver effective simulation to aspiring critical care nurses.

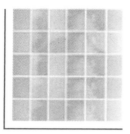

Acknowledgments

*W*e would like to acknowledge Elizabeth Nieginski for her vision, dedication and ongoing support of this project. We would also like to acknowledge the professionalism and dedication of John Jordan, Eric Van Osten and all of the team at LWW in helping make this project a reality.

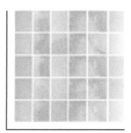

Contents

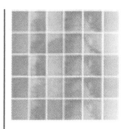

Chapter 1
Myocardial Infarction Case 1.0

At the completion of this case, the student will:

1. Recognize normal and abnormal assessment findings in the patient experiencing myocardial infarction (MI).
2. Prioritize interventions based on findings and assessments in the patient experiencing MI.
3. Be able to systematically interpret a 12-lead electrocardiogram (ECG) and discuss implications for a 15-lead ECG.
4. Demonstrate ability to systematically analyze arrhythmias.
5. Identify indications, contraindications, and side effects associated with cardiac pharmacological interventions.
6. Discuss anticipated treatment for life-threatening arrhythmias according to the current advanced cardiac life support (ACLS) guidelines.

Before viewing the video, Myocardial Infarction Case 1.0, complete the following five questions to help prepare you for the subsequent questions post-video and/or before attending the simulation lab.

1. Analyze the following 12-Lead ECG using the systematic approach for 12 leads as shown below.

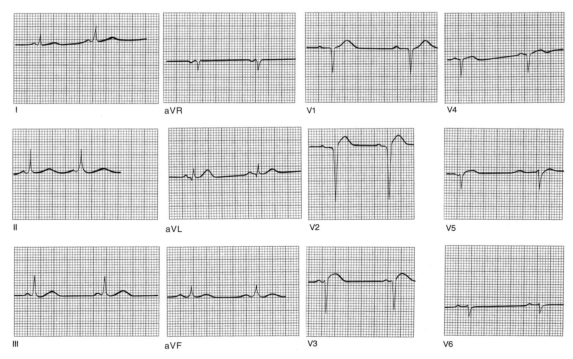

Systematic Approach: 12-Lead ECG Interpretation

Step	Approach
1	Analyze rhythm
2	Identify axis
3	Voltage (in precordial leads, limb leads)
4	R-wave progression (also, does transition occur at V3 or V4?)
5	Is there a bundle branch block?
6	Atrial or ventricular hypertrophy?
7	Analyze ST and T-wave changes. Is there a suspected MI present?
8	What stage is the MI at? (hyperacute or new, acute or old)

Response

Step	Answer
1	
2	
3	
4	
5	
6	
7	
8	

2. The nitroglycerine drip 50 mg/250 ml 5% dextrose in water (D5W) your patient is infusing has been titrated to 100 mcg/minute. What would be the correct rate to set the intravenous pump at?

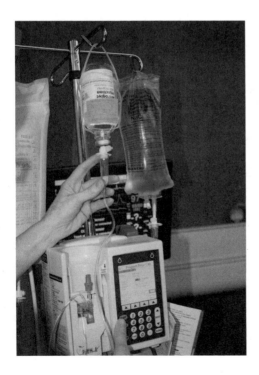

Answer:

_____

_____

_____

_____

_____

_____

3. Analyze the following two arrhythmias and compare and contrast the similarities and differences in presentation, significance, and anticipated treatment.

Strip 8-64. Rhythm:_____ Rate: _____ P wave: _____

PR interval: _____ QRS complex:_____

Rhythm interpretation: _____

Strip 8-71. Rhythm:_____ Rate: _____ P wave: _____

PR interval: _____ QRS complex:_____

Rhythm interpretation: _____

Answer:

_____

_____

_____

_____

_____

_____

4. One of the complications of an MI is cardiogenic shock. In the patient experiencing cardiogenic shock, it would be expected that the systemic vascular resistance (SVR), right atrial pressure (RAP), and wedge (pulmonary artery occlusion pressure; PAOP) would be increased, decreased, or remain normal? Why?

Answer:

_____

_____

_____

_____

_____

_____

5. Describe indications and placement of electrodes for a 15-lead ECG.

Answer:

_____

_____

_____

_____

_____

_____

_____

▼ POST-VIDEO OR -SIMULATION LAB

After watching the video and/or attending the simulation lab for this case, answer the following questions.

Scene

1. Describe the anticipated treatment for third-degree heart block.

Answer:

_____

_____

_____

_____

_____

2. Describe your treatment priorities once the patient became unstable.

Answer:

_____

_____

_____

_____

_____

3. The dopamine infusion 400 mg/250 ml D5W was infusing at 30 ml/hour. Calculate the infusion rate in mcg/kg/minute. (Patient weight is 100 kg)

Answer:

_____
_____
_____
_____
_____
_____

4. Click on the link for _lab values Colin Hawkins_ and discuss any abnormal values in addition to anticipated lab value changes in the patient experiencing an acute MI.

Answer:

_____
_____
_____
_____
_____
_____

5. Describe anticipated treatment should the patient have proceeded into asystole versus pulseless electrical activity (PEA).

Answer:

_____
_____
_____
_____
_____
_____

▼ SUGGESTED READINGS

American Heart Association (AHA). (2010). ACLS guidelines. _Circulation, 122_(18 Suppl 3), S640–S656.

Baird, M. S., & Bethel, S. (2011). _Manual of critical care nursing: Nursing interventions and collaborative management._ St. Louis, MO: Elsevier.

Fischbach, F., & Dunning, M. (2009). _A manual of laboratory and diagnostic tests._ Philadelphia, PA: Lippincott Williams & Wilkins.

Morton, P., & Fontaine, D. (2009). _Critical care nursing: A holistic approach._ Philadelphia, PA: Lippincott Williams & Wilkins.

Susala, G., Suffredini, A., McAreavey, D., Solomon, M., Hoffman, W., Nyquist, P., . . . Masur, H. (2006). _Handbook of critical care drug therapy._ Philadelphia, PA: Lippincott Williams & Wilkins.

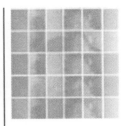

Chapter 2
Hypovolemic Shock Case 2.0

▼ **LEARNING OUTCOMES**

At the completion of this case, the student will:

1. Recognize normal and abnormal assessment findings in the patient experiencing hypovolemic shock.
2. Prioritize interventions based on findings and assessments.
3. Discuss principles of safe blood product administration.
4. Recognize signs and symptoms of hypovolemic shock.
5. Discuss potential signs and describe treatment of transfusion reactions in addition to risks associated with multiple transfusions.
6. Demonstrate ability to analyze arrhythmias and intervene appropriately.
7. Identify indications, contraindications, and side effects associated with interventions in the patient experiencing hypovolemic shock.
8. Identify accurate treatment of life-threatening arrhythmias according to the advanced cardiac life support (ACLS) current guidelines.

▼ **PREPARING FOR SIMULATION**

Before viewing the video, Hypovolemic Shock Case 2.0, complete the following five questions to help prepare you for the subsequent questions post-video and/or before attending the simulation lab.

1. Complete the following table relating to a hemodynamic profile of a patient experiencing hypovolemic shock. Indicate whether the value would be increased (↑), decreased (↓), or remain normal (N).

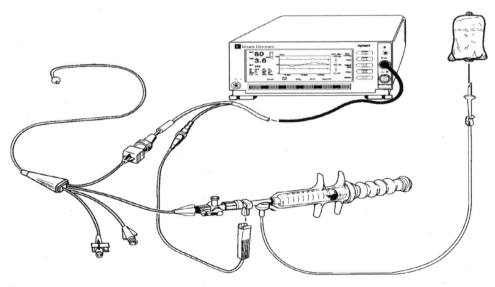

Hemodynamic Profile: Hypovolemic Shock

	Expected Change: Increased (↑), Decreased (↓), or Normal (N)
Cardiac output (C.O.)	
Cardiac index (C.I.)	
Heart rate	
Mean arterial pressure (MAP)	
Pulmonary artery pressure (PAP)	
Systemic vascular resistance (SVR)	
Pulmonary vascular resistance (PVR)	
Pulmonary artery occlusive pressure (PAOP)	
Right atrial pressure (RAP)	
Left ventricular stroke work Index (LVSWI)	
Right ventricular stroke work Index (RVSWI)	

TIP: this would be an excellent cue card/download for practice in the ICU or simulation lab. See Appendixxx for details.

2. What are the risks for patients with multiple transfusions?

Answer:

_____

_____

_____

_____

_____

_____

3. What other blood products may be considered for administration once multiple units of packed cells have been transfused?

Answer:

_____

_____

_____

_____

_____

_____

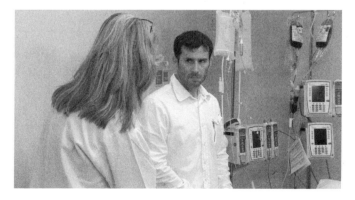

4. In the patient experiencing hypovolemic shock, should fluids or inotropes be administered initially? Why?

Answer:

_____

_____

_____

_____

_____

_____

5. The intravenous solution of choice for treatment of hypovolemic shock is
   a) Hypotonic crystalloid
   b) Colloid
   c) Hypertonic crystalloid
   d) Isotonic crystalloid

▼ POST-VIDEO OR -SIMULATION LAB

After watching the video and/or attending the simulation lab for this case, answer the following questions:

Scene 1

1. Discuss the algorithm for pulseless ventricular tachycardia.

Answer:

_____

_____

_____

_____

_____

_____

2. Contrast the ventricular tachycardia and pulseless electrical activity (PEA) algorithm.

Answer:

_____

_____

_____

_____

_____

_____

3. The most likely cause of Mrs. Chu's cardiac arrest was
   a) Coronary thrombosis
   b) Tension pneumothorax
   c) Hypovolemia
   d) Hyperkalemia

After watching Scene 2, answer the following questions.

4. What signs and symptoms (red flags) would you be assessing for to indicate Mrs. Chu's condition is worsening?

Answer:

_____

_____

_____

_____

_____

_____

5. Describe how you would support Mrs. Chu's husband and what resources would you advocate for?

Answer:

_____

_____

_____

_____

_____

_____

▼ SUGGESTED READINGS

American Heart Association. (2010). ACLS guidelines. *Circulation, 122*(18 Suppl 3), S640–S656.

Baird, M. S., & Bethel, S (2011). *Manual of critical care nursing: Nursing interventions and collaborative management.* St. Louis, MO: Elsevier.

Fischbach, F., & Dunning, M. (2009). *A manual of laboratory and diagnostic tests.* Philadelphia, PA: Lippincott Williams & Wilkins.

Morton, P., & Fontaine, D. (2009). *Critical care nursing: A holistic approach.* Philadelphia, PA: Lippincott Williams & Wilkins.

Strickler, J. (2010). Traumatic hypovolemic shock: Halting the downward spiral. *Nursing, 40*(10), 34–39.

Susala, G., Suffredini, A., McAreavey, D., Solomon, M., Hoffman, W., Nyquist, P., . . . Masur, H. (2006). *Critical care drug therapy.* Philadelphia, PA: Lippincott Williams & Wilkins.

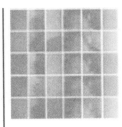

Chapter 3
Abdominal Aortic Aneurysm Repair Case 3.0

At the completion of this case, the student will:

1. Recognize normal and abnormal assessment findings.
2. Prioritize interventions based on findings and assessments.
3. Document assessment findings.
4. Analyze and interpret arterial and pulmonary artery waveforms.
5. Identify postoperative complications such as limb ischemia.
6. Demonstrate ability to analyze arrhythmias and intervene appropriately.
7. Administer medications accurately and identify indications, contraindications, and side effects associated with interventions.
8. Initiate ABC primary survey, administer volume as indicated, manage postoperative pain, and trouble-shoot ventilator.
9. Describe nursing management of a surgical patient in the immediate postoperative phase.

Before viewing the video, Abdominal Aortic Aneurysm Repair Case 3.0, complete the following five questions to help prepare you for the subsequent questions post-video and/or before attending the simulation lab.

1. Analyze the following hemodynamic profile including the anticipated nursing interventions for a patient returning to the intensive care unit after an abdominal aortic aneurysm repair. Indicate whether the value increased, decreased, or remained normal.

Measure	Value	Increased (↑), Decreased (↓), or Normal (N)
Cardiac output (C.O.)	6 L/min	
Cardiac index (C.I.)	2.5 L/min/m²	
Heart rate	135 beats/min	
Temperature	95.6°F (35°C)	
Mean arterial pressure (MAP)	61 mmHg	
Pulmonary artery pressure (PAP)	22/12 mmHg	
Systemic vascular resistance (SVR)	1700 dynes/sec/cm^{-5}	
Pulmonary vascular resistance (PVR)	250 dynes/sec/cm^{-5}	
Pulmonary artery occlusive pressure (PAOP)	10 mmHg	
Right atrial pressure (RAP)	6 mmHg	
Left ventricular stroke work index (LVSWI)	45 g-m/m²	
Right ventricular stroke work index (RVSWI)	7 g-m/m²	

Interpretation:_____

Anticipated nursing interventions:

a._____

b._____

2. The patient has a propofol infusion for sedation during mechanical ventilation. This infusion is supplied in 50 ml premixed bottles at 10 mg/ml. The pump is set at 10.5 ml/hour. How much propofol is the patient receiving? The patient weighs 70 kg.

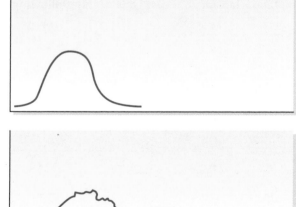

Answer:

_____

_____

_____

_____

_____

_____

3. Compare and contrast the cardiac output curves below. Be sure to include key steps to ensure accuracy in performing cardiac outputs.

Answer:

_____
_____
_____
_____
_____
_____

4. Identify the immediate postoperative nursing/collaborative priorities when caring for a patient undergoing an abdominal aortic aneurysm repair. Include rationale.

Answer:

_____
_____
_____
_____
_____
_____

5. Describe the six signs of poor arterial perfusion.

Answer:

_____
_____
_____
_____
_____
_____

▼ POST-VIDEO OR -SIMULATION LAB

After watching the video and/or attending the simulation lab for this case, answer the following questions.

Scene 1

6. Describe hemodynamic consequences of atrial fibrillation.

Answer:

_____
_____
_____
_____
_____

7. Describe your treatment priorities once Laura Lewis begins to emerge from anesthesia after an abdominal aortic aneurysm (AAA) repair; include at least one nursing intervention for each.

Answer:

_____

_____

_____

_____

_____

_____

8. Important communication is shared between the OR health care team and the critical care nurse. List the elements of a comprehensive handover report for a postoperative patient.

Answer: (Minimum 8)

_____

_____

_____

_____

_____

_____

9. What is the best nursing action to prevent pressure on the surgical site after an AAA repair during the first 72 hours postoperative phase? (Circle all that apply)
a) Encourage patient to lie in supine position
b) Elevate head of bed (HOB) no greater than 30° to 45°
c) Place in high fowlers position
d) Mobilize from lying to standing, avoiding sitting position

10. Describe anticipated treatment for Laura Lewis postoperative AAA repair, when the monitor displays the following:

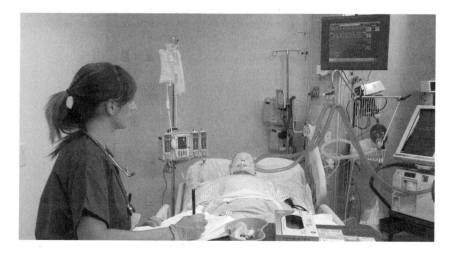

Lead II
HR 150

BP 85/50 mmHg	PVR 200 dynes/sec/cm^{-2}
PAP 20/10 mmHg	SVR 1850 dynes/sec/cm^{-2}
PAOP 8 mmHg	CO 5 L/min
CVP 4 mmHg	CI 1.8 L/min/m^2

Answer:

_____

_____

_____

_____

_____

_____

▼ SUGGESTED READINGS

Bickley, L., & Szilagyi, P. (2009). *Bates' guide to physical examination and history taking* (10th ed.). Philadelphia, PA: Lippincott Williams & Wilkins (Chap. 12).

Diehl, T. (Ed) (2011). *ECG Interpretation made incredibly easy.* (5th ed., Chapter 5) Philadelphia: Lippincott Williams & Wilkins.

Karch, A. (2011). *Lippincott's nursing drug guide.* Philadelphia, PA: Lippincott Williams & Wilkins.

Morton, P., & Fontaine, D. (2010). Chapters 13, 17, 19. In *Critical care nursing: A holistic approach* (9th ed.). Philadelphia, PA: Lippincott Williams & Wilkins.

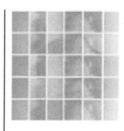

Chapter 4
Closed Head Injury Case 4.0

At the completion of this case, the student will:

1. Recognize normal and abnormal assessment findings.
2. Prioritize interventions based on findings and assessments.
3. Document assessment findings.
4. Demonstrate nursing management of a patient experiencing a closed head injury.
5. Demonstrate ability to analyze dysrhythmias and intervene appropriately.
6. Administer medications accurately and identify indications, contraindications, and side effects associated with interventions.
7. Initiate ABC primary survey, identifying key priorities to decrease intracranial pressure (ICP).

▼ PREPARING FOR SIMULATION

Before viewing the video, Closed Head Injury Case 4.0, complete the following five questions to help prepare you for the subsequent questions post-video and/or before attending the simulation lab.

1. Identify causes of increased ICP in a patient with a closed head injury, including the nursing management.

Causes of Increased ICP	Nursing Management

2. Early signs of increased ICP include: (Circle best answer)

a) Alteration in BP and HR
b) Alteration in level of consciousness
c) Fixed and dilated pupils
d) Irregular respiratory rate

3. Review the following motor responses to pain. Indicate which figure represents the most extensive brain injury?

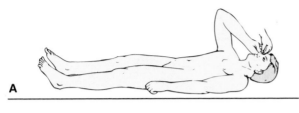

A

(A) Localizing pain. An appropriate response is to reach up above shoulder level toward the stimulus. Remember, a focal motor deficit such as hemiplegia may prevent a bilateral response.

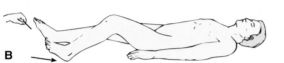

B

(B) Withdrawal. An appropriate response is to pull the extremity or body away from the stimulus. As brainstem involvement increases, your patient may respond by assuming one of the following postures. Each one shows more advanced deterioration.

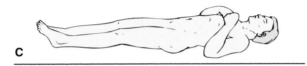

C

(C) Decorticate posturing. One or both arms in full flexion on the chest. Legs may be stiffly extended.

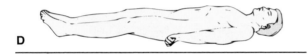

D

(D) Decerebrate posturing. One or both arms stiffly extended. Possible extension of the legs.

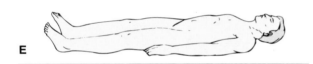

E

(E) Flaccid. No motor response in any extremity.

a) *(localizing to pain)*
b) *(withdrawal to pain)*
c) *(decorticate posturing*
d) *(decerebrate posturing)*

4. The patient with a closed head injury was admitted without analgesic orders written. How would the nurse advocate for the patient? Include rationale.

Answer:

_____

_____

_____

_____

_____

_____

5. List the priority assessments for a patient experiencing a closed head injury.

Answer:

_____

_____

_____

_____

_____

_____

▼ POST-VIDEO OR -SIMULATION LAB

After watching the video and/or attending the simulation lab for this case, answer the following questions.

Scene 2

1. Martin Neylander required temporary transcutaneous pacing for second-degree AB block Type II. The alarm on the bedside monitor rings for the following:

Describe the nurse's priority actions.

Answer:

_____

_____

_____

_____

_____

_____

2. The cerebral perfusion pressure (CPP) is dependent on an adequate mean arterial pressure (MAP): CPP = MAP − ICP. List medications that may be ordered to promote adequate cerebral perfusion; include rationale.

Answer:

_____

_____

_____

_____

_____

_____

3. Martin Neylander is at high risk for experiencing a seizure. If Martin should experience a generalized seizure involving tonic–clonic movement of all extremities, describe nursing management.

Answer:

_____

_____

_____

_____

_____

_____

4. Enteral feeds were commenced for Martin Neylander via oral gastric tube. The nurse from the earlier shift reported that he had hypoactive bowel sounds and abdominal distension was noted. Upon present assessment, the nurse notes that Martin has high gastric residual volumes (i.e., 400 ml aspirated). What is the next step for the nurse to perform?

a) Report to the dietician
b) Hold feeds for 1 to 2 hours and reassess
c) Continue feeds and reassess in 4 hours
d) Bolus feedings every 4 hours

5. After watching Scene 2, explain the rationale for the nurse advocating for a head CT scan for Martin.

Answer:

_____

_____

_____

_____

_____

_____

▼ SUGGESTED READINGS

American Heart Association. (2010). 2010 American Heart Association guidelines for cardiopulmonary resuscitation and emergency cardiovascular care. *Circulation, 122*(Suppl. 3), S746–S756.

Bickley, L. (2009). Chapter 17. In *Bates' guide to physical assessment and history taking* (10th ed.). Philadelphia, PA: Lippincott Williams & Wilkins.

Diepenbrock, N. (2012). Chapter 1. In *Quick reference to critical care* (4th ed). Philadelphia, PA: Lippincott Williams & Wilkins.

Hickey, J. (2009). Chapter 17. In *The clinical practice of neurological & neurosurgical nursing* (6th ed.). Philadelphia, PA: Lippincott Williams & Wilkins.

Karch, A. (2011). *Lippincott's nursing drug guide.* Philadelphia, PA: Lippincott Williams & Wilkins.

Morton, P., & Fontaine, D. (2010). Chapters 32, 33, 34, & 36. In *Critical care nursing: A holistic approach* (9th ed.). Philadelphia, PA: Lippincott Williams & Wilkins.

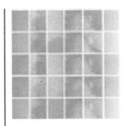

Chapter 5
Adult Respiratory Distress Syndrome (ARDS) Case 5.0

At the completion of this case, the student will:

1. Recognize normal and abnormal assessment findings in the patient experiencing adult respiratory distress syndrome (ARDS).
2. Identify worsening patient condition and anticipate likely interventions for ARDS.
3. Identify indications, contraindications, and side effects associated with pharmacological and diagnostic interventions.
4. Accurately interpret arterial blood gas (ABG) results.
5. Discuss safe management of patient receiving neuromuscular blocking agents.
6. Demonstrate ability to troubleshoot mechanical ventilator alarms and suggest adjustments as appropriate.

Before viewing the video, ARDS Case 5.0, complete the following five questions to help prepare you for the subsequent questions post-video and/or before attending the simulation lab.

1. Compare and contrast volume modes of ventilation (i.e., synchronized intermittent mandatory ventilation; SIMV) with pressure control modes (i.e., pressure controlled ventilation; PCV) and include advantages and disadvantages of each.

Answer:

_____

_____

_____

_____

_____

_____

2. Interpret the following ABG results and describe anticipated treatments.

   a) pH 7.30
   b) pCO_2 58
   c) HCO_3^- 29
   d) PO_2 70

   Tip: use the ABG systematic approach found in Appendix D.

Answer:

_____
_____
_____
_____
_____
_____

3. One of the care priorities in the patient experiencing ARDS is to reduce the tidal volume to 4 to 6 ml/kg. Why?

Answer:

_____
_____
_____
_____
_____
_____

4. Describe one of the complications of ARDS and associated signs and symptoms.

Answer:

_____
_____
_____
_____
_____
_____

5. Describe risk factors for ARDS.

Answer:

_____
_____
_____
_____
_____
_____

▼ POST-VIDEO OR -SIMULATION LAB

After watching the video and/or attending the simulation lab for this case, answer the following questions.

1. Describe the anticipated treatment for ARDS.

Answer:

_____

_____

_____

_____

_____

_____

2. After watching the video, discuss the signs and symptoms ("red flags") you observed or would anticipate that would indicate the patient's condition is worsening.

Answer:

_____

_____

_____

_____

_____

_____

3. The ventilator alarms were frequently alarming "high pressure" in the scenario. What is the likely cause of this and what would your priority interventions be?

Answer:

_____

_____

_____

_____

_____

_____

4. Click on link for _Mr. Townsend's lab values_ and discuss any abnormal values as well as changes that may be anticipated as his condition deteriorates.

Answer:

_____

_____

_____

_____

_____

_____

5. At the end of the scenario in the handover report, it was suggested that the patient may be placed on neuromuscular blockade. Why do you think this may be ordered and what safety precautions must be considered in the patient receiving neuromuscular blockade?

Answer:

_____

_____

_____

_____

_____

_____

▼ SUGGESTED READINGS

Baird, M. S., & Bethel, S. (2011). *Manual of critical care nursing: Nursing interventions and collaborative management.* St. Louis, MO: Elsevier.

Fischbach, F., & Dunning, M. (2009). *A manual of laboratory and diagnostic tests.* Philadelphia, PA: Lippincott Williams & Wilkins.

Morton, P., & Fontaine, D. (2009). *Critical care nursing: A holistic approach.* Philadelphia, PA: Lippincott Williams & Wilkins.

Susala, G., Suffredini, A., McAreavey, D., Solomon, M., Hoffman, W., Nyquist, P., . . . Masur, H. (2006). *Handbook of critical care drug therapy.* Philadelphia, PA: Lippincott Williams & Wilkins.

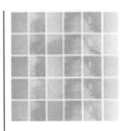

Chapter 6
Renal Failure Case 6.0

At the completion of this case, the student will:

1. Recognize normal and abnormal assessment findings.
2. Prioritize interventions based on findings and assessments.
3. Document assessment findings.
4. Demonstrate accurate management of hemodynamic lines.
5. Demonstrate ability to systematically interpret arrhythmias as related to patient condition.
6. Demonstrate ability to analyze lab data and integrate with patient assessment.
7. Administer medications accurately and can identify indications, contraindications, and side effects associated with interventions.

Before viewing the video, Renal Failure Case 6.0, complete the following five questions to help prepare you for the subsequent questions post-video and/or before attending the simulation lab.

1. Analyze the following hemodynamic profile including the anticipated nursing interventions for a patient postoperative day 3 after a quadruple coronary artery bypass. Indicate whether the value is increased, decreased, or normal.

Measure	Value	Increased (↑), Decreased (↓), or Normal (N)
Cardiac output (C.O.)	4 L/min	
Cardiac index (C.I.)	2.2 L/min/m^2	
Heart rate	110 beats/min	
Temperature	F 95.6°F (37°C)	
Mean arterial pressure (MAP)	61 mmHg	
Pulmonary arterial pressure (PAP)	35/18 mmHg	
Systemic vascular resistance (SVR)	1484 dynes/sec/cm^{-5}	
Pulmonary vascular resistance (PVR)	325 dynes/sec/cm^{-5}	
Pulmonary artery occlusion pressure (PAOP)	17 mmHg	
Right atrial pressure (RAP)	12 mmHg	
Left ventricular stroke eork index (LVSWI)	41 g-m/m^2	
Right ventricular stroke work index (RVSWI)	9 g-m/m^2	

Interpretation:_____

Anticipated nursing interventions:

  a)_____

  b)_____

2. List the clinical manifestations of hyperkalemia. Review the rhythm strip below and list the clinical manifestations of hyperkalemia.

Answer:

_____

_____

_____

_____

_____

_____

3. What is the key priority in nursing management of a patient experiencing diabetic ketoacidosis? (Circle the best answer)
   a) Oral care to eliminate fruity breath or acetone odor
   b) Replacement (as ordered) for hypovolemia/hyperosmolality
   c) Reduce and normalize glucose levels quickly
   d) Assess for signs of infection

4. Describe conditions that put the patient at a higher risk of renal failure.

Answer:

_____

_____

_____

_____

_____

_____

5. Define the term anion gap.

Answer:

_____

_____

_____

_____

_____

_____

▼ POST-VIDEO OR -SIMULATION LAB

After watching the video and/or attending the simulation lab for this case, answer the following questions.

Scene 2

1. Compare and contrast defibrillation and cardioversion.

Answer:

_____

_____

_____

_____

_____

_____

2. Identify the reasons Anthony Liu experienced supraventricular tachycardia.

Answer:

_____

_____

_____

_____

_____

_____

3. What factors contributed to Anthony Liu developing renal failure? (Circle the best answer)

    a) Decreased cardiac output during surgery
    b) Drug toxicity
    c) Renal calculi
    d) Cystitis

4. Identify four nursing considerations when caring for Anthony Liu in acute renal failure.

Answer:

_____

_____

_____

_____

_____

5. Describe indications for continuous renal replacement therapy (CRRT).

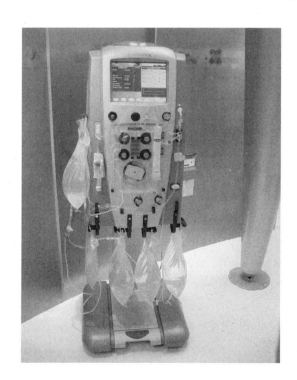

Answer:

_____

_____

_____

_____

_____

_____

▼ SUGGESTED READINGS

Bickley, L., & Szilagyi, P. (2009). *Bates' guide to physical examination and history taking* (10th ed.). Philadelphia, PA: Lippincott, Williams & Wilkins.

Diepenbrock, N. (2012). *Quick reference to critical care* (4th ed.). Philadelphia, PA: Lippincott, Williams & Wilkins.

Karch, A. (2011). *Lippincott's nursing drug guide*. Philadelphia, PA: Lippincott Williams & Wilkins.

LWW. (2010). *ECG interpretation: An incredibly easy pocket guide* (2nd ed., pp. 140–142). Philadelphia, PA: Lippincott, Williams & Wilkins.

Morton, P., & Fontaine, D. (2009). *Critical care nursing: A holistic approach* (9th ed.). Philadelphia, PA: Lippincott, Williams & Wilkins.

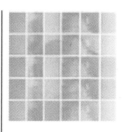

Chapter 7
Liver Failure Case 7.0

At the completion of this case, the student will:

1. Recognize normal and abnormal assessment findings in the patient experiencing liver failure.
2. Recognize abnormal lab values related to liver failure.
3. Prioritize interventions based on findings and assessments in the patient experiencing liver failure.
4. Describe complications associated with liver failure.
5. Discuss rationale for medications and diagnostics ordered in the patient experiencing acute liver failure.
6. Reflect on the use of advanced communication skills and ethical considerations in an end of life family conference.

▼ PREPARING FOR SIMULATION

Before viewing the video, Liver Failure Case 7.0, complete the following five questions to help prepare you for the subsequent questions post-video and/or before attending the simulation lab.

1. What lab values are essential to evaluate in the patient experiencing liver failure?

Answer:

_____
_____
_____
_____
_____
_____

2. What gastrointestinal findings would the nurse anticipate on assessment of the patient?

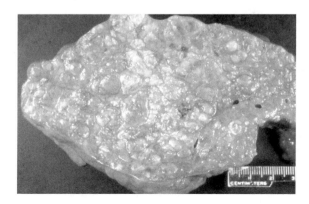

Answer:

_____

_____

_____

_____

_____

_____

3. In the patient experiencing end stage liver failure secondary to alcoholic cirrhosis, what complication could lead to hepatic encephalopathy?

   a) Hypoalbuminemia
   b) Gastrointestinal bleeding
   c) Splenomegaly
   d) Hypercholesteremia

4. What are the signs that your patient is progressing into hepatic coma or the hepatic encephalopathy is worsening?

Answer:

_____

_____

_____

_____

_____

_____

5. Liver biopsy is often ordered in liver failure to monitor the stage of the disease. What precautions should be taken post-biopsy? Why?

Answer:

_____

_____

_____

_____

_____

_____

▼ POST-VIDEO OR -SIMULATION LAB

After watching the video and/or attending the simulation lab for this case, answer the following questions.

Scene 1

1. What information received in the initial handover report described the signs and symptoms specifically related to liver failure that you would expect to observe upon assessment of the patient?

Answer:

_____
_____
_____
_____
_____
_____

Scene 2

2. What is the significance of the rising serum ammonia (NH_3) level in Mr. Adams' case?

Answer:

_____
_____
_____
_____
_____
_____

3. What signs or symptoms would you anticipate to indicate Mr. Adams' condition is worsening?

Answer:

_____
_____
_____
_____
_____
_____

4. In identifying care priorities in the patient experiencing liver failure, the critical care nurse knows that all of the following interventions are a priority EXCEPT:

a) Sedatives should be avoided since they can precipitate or contribute to encephalopathy.
b) Sodium containing fluids are avoided to decrease cirrhosis ascites and reduce risk of renal insufficiency.
c) A high calorie, high protein diet is needed to decrease progression of hepatic encephalopathy.
d) Administration of vitamin K and fresh frozen plasma to prevent bleeding complications.

Scene 3: Confirm scene

5. After watching the scene in which the family conference takes place, describe the therapeutic communication techniques you observed being utilized. Think of a similar situation you may have had with a patient. What communication strategies were helpful? What would you do differently next time?

Answer:

_____

_____

_____

_____

_____

_____

▼ SUGGESTED READINGS

Baird, M. S., & Bethel, S. (2011). *Manual of critical care nursing: Nursing interventions and collaborative management.* St. Louis, MO: Elsevier.

Fischbach, F., & Dunning, M. (2009). *A manual of laboratory and diagnostic tests.* Philadelphia, PA: Lippincott Williams & Wilkins.

Morton, P., & Fontaine, D. (2009). *Critical care nursing: A holistic approach.* Philadelphia, PA: Lippincott Williams & Wilkins.

Susala, G., Suffredini, A., McAreavey, D., Solomon, M., Hoffman, W., Nyquist, P., . . . Masur, H. (2006). *Handbook of critical care drug therapy.* Philadelphia, PA: Lippincott Williams & Wilkins.

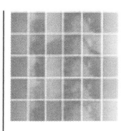

Chapter 8
Trauma Case 8.0

At the completion of this case, the student will:

1. Recognize normal and abnormal assessment findings.
2. Prioritize interventions based on findings and assessments.
3. Document assessment findings.
4. Demonstrate ability to manage chest drainage system.
5. Demonstrate ability to identify and prevent complications from multiple system trauma.
6. Administer medications accurately and identify indications, contraindications, and side effects associated with interventions.

Before viewing the video, Trauma Repair Case 8.0, complete the following five questions to help prepare you for the subsequent questions post-video and/or before attending the simulation lab.

1. Identify four common complications of multiple trauma and one nursing intervention to prevent the potential complication.

Answer:

_____

_____

_____

_____

_____

_____

2. Describe five components of the initial assessment of a patient with multiple trauma and provide a nursing intervention for each.

Answer:

_____

_____

_____

_____

_____

_____

3. What statement is correct about fat emboli? (Circle the best answer)
   a) Early use of low molecular weight heparin will prevent fat emboli
   b) Petechiae develop due to fat globules lodging in dermal capillaries
   c) A positive Homans' test will be noted
   d) Fat emboli syndrome can cause profuse bleeding

4. Identify a life-threatening condition and anticipated intervention for a patient with multiple fractured ribs. What would your assessment include?

Answer:

_____
_____
_____
_____
_____
_____

5. Explain how a patient with multiple trauma is at risk for compartment syndrome?

Answer:

_____
_____
_____
_____
_____
_____

▼ POST-VIDEO OR -SIMULATION LAB

After watching the video and/or attending the simulation lab for this case, answer the following questions.

Scene 2

1. After watching the video, how are Vijay Surrenda's BP and right atrial pressures being monitored? Please review the waveform below and identify nursing priorities.

Answer:

_____
_____
_____
_____
_____
_____

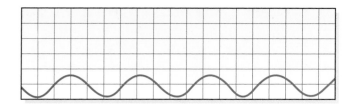

2. Vijay required intubation and mechanical ventilation due to respiratory distress. List four common ventilator alarms that may occur.

Answer:

_____

_____

_____

_____

_____

_____

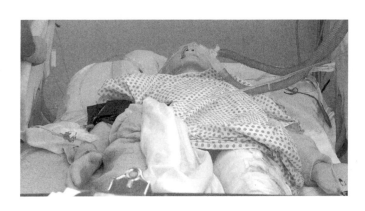

3. Vijay's family has just been notified of his motor vehicle collision and his condition. It is well past visiting hours, should the nurse violate the visiting hour policy and permit them to visit? Provide the rationale for your answer.

Answer:

_____

_____

_____

_____

_____

_____

4. Why is Vijay at high risk for a fat emboli?

    a) 12 to 36 hours after fractured long bones
    b) Smoking a pack of cigarettes per day
    c) Young men are more prone to fat emboli
    d) Dehydration due to lack of oral fluids

5. Vijay was ventilated for 72 hours and is now ready to wean. What weaning criteria are assessed to ensure Vijay is ready for extubation?

Answer:

_____

_____

_____

_____

_____

_____

▼ SUGGESTED READINGS

Bickley, L., & Szilagyi, P. (2009). *Bates' guide to physical examination and history taking* (10th ed., pp. 591–637, 296–309). Philadelphia, PA: Lippincott, Williams & Wilkins.

Critical care made incredibly easy. (2012). Philadelphia, PA: Lippincott, Williams & Wilkins.

Diepenbrock, N. (2012). *Quick reference to critical care* (4th ed., pp. 382–383). Philadelphia, PA: Lippincott Williams & Wilkins.

Gore, T., & Lacey, S. (2005) Bone up on fate embolism syndrome. *Nursing, 35*(8), 32hn1–32hn4.

Karch, A. (2011). *Lippincott's nursing drug guide.* Philadelphia, PA: Lippincott Williams & Wilkins.

Morton, P., & Fontaine, D. (2009). *Critical care nursing: A holistic approach* (9th ed., pp. 35, 1437–1453). Philadelphia, PA: Lippincott Williams & Wilkins.

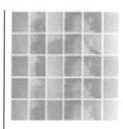

Chapter 9
Septic Shock Case 9.0

▼ **LEARNING OUTCOMES**

At the completion of this case, the student will be able to:

1. Recognize normal and abnormal assessment findings in septic shock.
2. Identify signs and symptoms of septic shock.
3. Prioritize interventions for septic shock based on findings and assessments.
4. Identify nursing management priorities of a patient in septic shock integrating the international guidelines for treatment of septic shock.
5. Identify indications, contraindications, and side effects associated with pharmacological therapy in septic shock.
6. Demonstrate ability to accurately calculate vasoactive drips.

▼ **PREPARING FOR SIMULATION**

Before viewing the video, Septic Shock 9.0, complete the following five questions to help prepare you for the subsequent questions post-video and/or before attending the simulation lab.

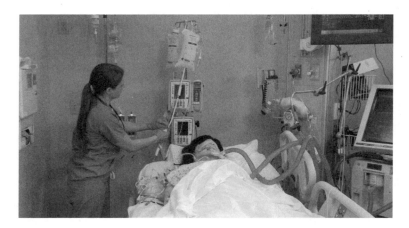

1. The norepinephrine intravenous (IV) infusion 4 mg/250 ml 5% dextrose in water (D5W) your patient is infusing has been titrated up to 4 mcg/minute. What would be the correct rate to set the IV pump at?

Answer:

_____

_____

_____

_____

_____

_____

Hemodynamic Profile: Septic Shock

2. Complete the following table for the patient experiencing septic shock.

	Expected Change: Increased (↑), Decreased (↓), or Normal (N)
Cardiac output (C.O.)	
Cardiac index (C.I.)	
Heart rate	
Mean arterial pressure (MAP)	
Pulmonary Arterial Pressure (PAP)	
Systemic vascular resistance (SVR)	
Pulmonary vascular resistance (PVR)	
Pulmonary artery occlusion pressure (PAOP)	
Right atrial pressure (RAP)	
Left ventricular stroke work index (LVSWI)	
Right ventricular stroke work index (RVSWI)	

3. List the seven key elements in the treatment of sepsis as outlined in the Surviving Sepsis Campaign International Guidelines.

Answer:

_____

_____

_____

_____

_____

_____

4. All of the following are considered essential components of early goal directed therapy in septic shock EXCEPT:
a) IV fluid resuscitation
b) IV vasodilator infusion
c) IV vasopressor infusion
d) Transfusion of packed red blood cells (RBCs)

5. Recombinant human activated protein C (rhAPC) has been shown in large trials to reduce mortality in patients with septic shock. What is one of the absolute contraindications to the administration of this treatment?

Answer:

_____

_____

_____

_____

_____

_____

▼ POST-VIDEO OR -SIMULATION LAB

After watching the video and/or attending the simulation lab for this case, answer the following questions.

Scene 1

1. From the handover report given, what signs and symptoms are indicative of septic shock in Mr. French?

Answer:

_____

_____

_____

_____

_____

_____

Scene 2

2. Describe your treatment priorities once the patient became unstable.

Answer:

_____

_____

_____

_____

_____

3. Click on the following link '*lab values John French*' and discuss the values that are abnormal and their relationship to septic shock.

Answer:

_____

_____

_____

_____

_____

_____

4. What signs or "red flags" would indicate to you that Mr. French's condition is worsening?

Answer:

_____

_____

_____

_____

_____

_____

5. Mr. French's dopamine infusion had to be titrated up to15 mcg/kg/minute in order to sustain his blood pressure. What is the maximum recommended dosage in mcg/kg/minute and what are the consequences to the patient with high dose dopamine administration?

Answer:

_____

_____

_____

_____

_____

_____

▼ SUGGESTED READINGS

Baird, M. S., & Bethel, S. (2011). *Manual of critical care nursing: Nursing interventions and collaborative management.* St Louis, MO: Elsevier.

Dellinger, R., Levy, M., & Carlet, J. (2008). Surviving sepsis campaign: International guidelines for management of severe sepsis and septic shock. Intensive Care Medicine, *34*, 17–60.

Morton, P., & Fontaine, D. (2009). *Critical care nursing: A holistic approach.* Philadelphia, PA: Lippincott Williams & Wilkins.

Susala, G., Suffredini, A., McAreavey, D., Solomon, M., Hoffman, W., Nyquist, P., . . . Masur, H. (2006). *Handbook of critical care drug therapy.* Philadelphia, PA: Lippincott Williams & Wilkins.

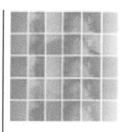

Chapter 10
Drug Overdose Case 10.0

At the completion of this case, the student will:

1. Recognize normal and abnormal assessment findings.
2. Prioritize interventions based on findings and assessments.
3. Document assessment findings.
4. Demonstrate ability to analyze arrhythmias and intervene appropriately.
5. Administer medications accurately and can identify indications, contraindications, and side effects associated with interventions.
6. Call for assistance of team as appropriate and initiate an intervention for a seizure.
7. Initiate a primary ABC survey and safely manage a general seizure.
8. Demonstrate ability to provide a concise, thorough hand-off report to the oncoming shift.

▼ PREPARING FOR SIMULATION

Before viewing the video, Drug Overdose Case 10.0, complete the following five questions to help prepare you for the subsequent questions post-video and/or before attending the simulation lab.

1. Analyze the following 12-lead ECG using the systematic approach for 12 leads as shown below.

Systematic Approach: 12 Lead ECG Interpretation

Step	Approach
1	
2	
3	
4	
5	
6	
7	
8	

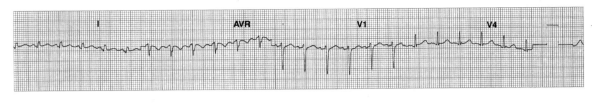

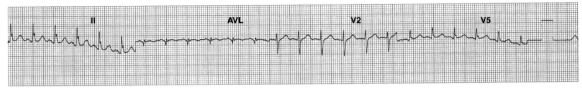

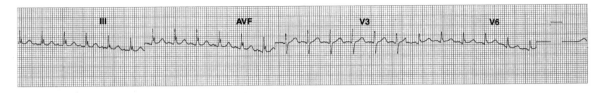

Response:

Step	Answer
1	
2	
3	
4	
5	
6	
7	
8	

2. Sodium bicarbonate is ordered for a tricyclic overdose to alkalinize the blood to minimize ventricular arrhythmias. What nursing actions are appropriate to ensure patient safety? (Circle the best answer)
   a) Administer via minibag over 15 to 20 minutes
   b) Use a filter to administer drug
   c) Keep protected from light
   d) Confirm patency of vein to avoid extravasation

3. Identify appropriate diagnostic tests ordered for patients ingesting an overdose of tricyclic antidepressants.

Answer:
_____
_____
_____
_____
_____
_____

4. Describe the cardiac effects of an overdose of tricyclic antidepressant medications.

Answer:

---

5. Explain priority treatment options ordered for ingestion of a drug overdose. Include rationale.

Answer:

▼ POST-VIDEO OR -SIMULATION LAB

After watching the video and/or attending the simulation lab for this case, answer the following questions.

Scene 2

1. Describe key nursing priorities when caring for Emily Jackson after ingesting an overdose of tricyclic antidepressants in a suicide attempt.

Answer:

---

2. Emily's airway is protected with a T-piece. Describe this method of oxygen delivery.

Answer:

---

3. Emily's monitor alarms for an idioventricular rhythm with a rate of 30 bpm. What is the priority?

Answer:

_____

_____

_____

_____

_____

_____

4. When Emily's mother visits her at the bedside, how would the nurse provide family centered care?

Answer:

_____

_____

_____

_____

_____

_____

5. After Emily has a generalized seizure, she is placed on the mechanical ventilator. Why does Emily require ventilator support at the present time? List all of the reasons.

Answers:

_____

_____

_____

_____

_____

_____

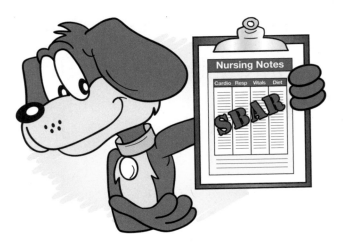

▼ SUGGESTED READINGS

Bickley, L., & Szilagyi, P. (2009). *Bates' guide to physical examination and history taking* (10th ed.). Philadelphia, PA: Lippincott Williams & Wilkins.

Diepenbrock, N. (2012). *Quick reference to critical care* (4th ed.). Philadelphia, PA: Lippincott Williams & Wilkins.

Karch, A. (2011). *Nursing drug guide*. Philadelphia, PA: Lippincott Williams & Wilkins.

Morton, P., & Fontaine, D. (2009). *Critical care nursing: A holistic approach* (9th ed.). Philadelphia, PA: Lippincott, Williams & Wilkins.

ICU/ER facts made incredibly easy. (2011). Philadelphia, PA.

Systematic Approach to Arrhythmia Interpretation

1. **Rhythm.** Is the rhythm regular or irregular? (p-p, R-R)

2. **Rate.** What is the rate?

3. **P waves.** Are the P waves uniform, upright, symmetrical, one for every QRS?

4. **pri.** Calculate the pri (normal is 0.12 to 0.20 seconds).

5. **QRS.** Calculate QRS interval (normal is 0.06 to 0.10 seconds).

6. **ST or T wave changes.** Assess for ST elevation or depression and changes in T wave (ie, inversion).

7. **Interpretation.** Name the rhythm.

8. **Nursing Management Priorities.**

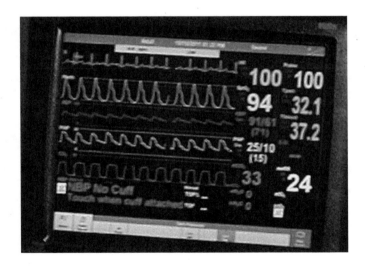

Appendix B

Systematic Approach: 12-Lead ECG Interpretation

Step	Approach
1	Analyze rhythm
2	Identify axis
3	Voltage (in precordial leads, limb leads)
4	R-wave progression (also does transition occur at V3 or V4?)
5	Is there a bundle branch block?
6	Atrial or ventricular hypertrophy?
7	Analyze ST and T-wave changes. Is there a suspected MI present?
8	What stage is the MI at? (hyperacute or new, acute or old)

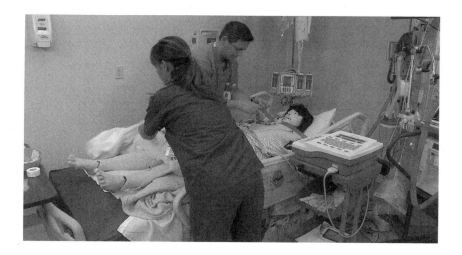

Vasoactive Drip Calculations

1. mcg/kg/minute to ml/hour:

$$\frac{\text{Weight (kg)} \times \text{dose ordered (mcg/kg/minute)} \times 60 \text{ (minute/hour)}}{\text{Concentration in bag (mcg/ml)}}$$

2. mg/minute to ml/hour:

$$\frac{\text{Dose ordered (mg/minute)} \times 60 \text{ (minute/hour)}}{\text{Concentration in bag (mg/ml)}}$$

3. ml/hour to mcg/kg/minute:

$$\frac{\text{Concentration in bag (mcg/ml)} \times \text{rate (ml/hour)}}{60 \text{ (minute/hour)} \times \text{weight (kg)}}$$

4. ml/hour to mg/minute:

$$\frac{\text{Concentration in bag (mg/ml)} \times \text{rate (ml/hour)}}{60 \text{ (minute/hour)}}$$

Arterial Blood Gas Interpretation

Step 1: Analyze all values (acidic, alkaline, normal)

Step 2: Which value matches ph (this helps determine whether it is a respiratory (CO_2) or metabolic issue (HCO_3^-) or both.)

Step 3: Determine whether there is compensation present (full, partial, none)

Step 4: Determine oxygenation issues by evaluating the PO_2 (ie, PO_2 80–100 mmHg, normal; PO_2 70–80 mmHg, mild hypoxemia; PO_2 60–70 mmHg, moderate hypoxemia; PO_2 < 60 mmHg, severe hypoxemia).

Example:

pH 7.33

PCO_2 58

HCO_3 28

PO_2 72

Step 1

pH and PCO_2 both acidic, HCO_3 alkalotic, PO_2 decreased.

Step 2

PCO_2 matches the pH, both are acidic therefore it is a respiratory acidosis.

Step 3

The HCO_3 is increased (more alkaline), therefore it is partially compensating. To have full compensation the pH would have had to return to normal.

Step 4

The PO_2 is 72 therefore there is mild hypoxemia present.

Interpretation: Respiratory acidosis with partial compensation and mild hypoxemia.

Pulmonary Artery Waveforms

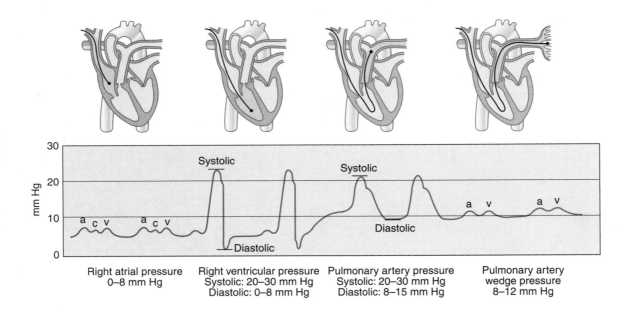

| Right atrial pressure
0–8 mm Hg | Right ventricular pressure
Systolic: 20–30 mm Hg
Diastolic: 0–8 mm Hg | Pulmonary artery pressure
Systolic: 20–30 mm Hg
Diastolic: 8–15 mm Hg | Pulmonary artery
wedge pressure
8–12 mm Hg |

**Red Flag Alert
*if catheter falls back into *right ventricle* the patient may experience ventricular dysrhythmias
*if catheter migrates forward into a spontaneous *wedge* position the patient may experience pulmonary infarction

Critical Care Pharmacology

Medication	Preparation	Dose	Key Nursing Considerations
Amiodarone (Cordarone)	900 mg/500 ml D_5W	150 mg/10 min, then 360 mg over 6 h; then 540 mg over 18 h	Use filter, mix in glass bottle, may prolong QT interval, monitor for hypotension and bradycardia
Dobutrex (Dobutamine)	250 mg/250 ml D_5W	2 to 20 mcg/kg/mg	Hypovolemia corrected first
Inotropin (Dopamine)	400 mg/250 ml D_5W	2–20 mcg/kg/min	Monitor for tachycardia and dysrhythmias, extravasation can cause sloughing
Epinephrine (Adrenaline)	1 mg/250 ml D_5W	1–10 mcg/min	↑ Myocardial oxygen demands
Levophed (Norepinephrine)	4 mg/250 ml D_5W	2–20 mcg/min	↑ Myocardial oxygen demands, extravasation can cause sloughing, monitor for ventricular tachycardia, and ventricular fibrillation
Nipride (Nitroprusside)	50 mg/500 ml D_5W	0.5–0 mcg/kg/min	Reconstitute with 3 ml D_5W, shield from light, observe for hypotension and thiocynate toxicity
Nitroglycerin (Nitroglycerin)	25 mg/250 ml/D_5W	5–200 mcg/kg/min	Use glass bottle, observe for tolerance, monitor for hypotension and bradycardia
Propofol (Diprivan)	10 mg/ml in 50 ml or 100 ml premixed	25–75 mcg/kg/min	Change tubing/vial every 12 hours, colors urine green, monitor for hypotension

**Follow institutional policy.
Karch, A. (2011). Lippincott's Nursing Drug Guide. Lippincott Williams & Wilkins.

Abnormal Lab Values and Assessment Findings

Red Flag Lab Values

	Lab Value	Assessment	Interventions
Hyponatremia	<135 mEq/L	Nausea and vomiting, weakness, irritability, seizures, hypotension, tachycardia, coma	Restrict fluid intake, oral sodium supplements, sodium rich foods
Hyperatremia	>145 mEq/L	Agitation, thirst, hypertension, fever hyperreflexia restlessness, decreased level of consciousness	Discontinue medications that may cause hypernatremia, ie, ticarcillin, PO or IV fluid replacement, restrict sodium intake
Hypokalemia	<3.5 mEq/L	Hypotension, dysrhythmias, cardiac/respiratory arrest, paralytic ileus, muscle weakness, fatigue	Remove underlying cause, ie, diuretics, potassium supplementation (PO/IV), potassium rich foods
Hyperkalemia	>5 mEq/L	Tachycardia→bradycardia, nausea vomiting, flaccid paralysis, cardiac arrest	Closely monitor patients at risk (patients with acidosis, renal failure), remove underlying cause, i.e., angiotensin-converting enzyme inhibitor, administer loop diuretic, cation-exchange resin, ie, kayexalate, calcium gluconate or calcium chloride, sodium bicarbonate, regular insulin + hypertonic dextrose (D50W), hemodialysis Note: Level may be falsely elevated due to hemolysis of specimen; repeat test to confirm
Hypocalcemia	<8.5 mg/dl	Anxiety, laryngospasm, seizures, hypotension, dysrhythmias, positive Chvostek's and Trousseau's signs	IV calcium, if not responding to treatment add vitamin D supplements, oral calcium, foods rich in calcium
Hypercalcemia	10.1 mg/dl	Drowsiness, muscle flaccidity, headaches, bone pain and fractures, tingling in finger tips, seizures, heart block, cardiac arrest, ileus	Decrease dietary sources, stop Vitamin D supplements, loop diuretics, hydration with NS, medications to block bone reabsorption, ie, corticosteroids

(Continued)

	Lab Value	**Assessment**	**Interventions**
Hypomagnesemia	<1.5 mEq/L	Tetany, foot cramps, seizures, dysrhythmias, ie, supraventricular tachycardia, ventricular fibrillation positive Chovostek's and Trousseau sign	Encourage dietary sources, ie, bran, supplementation (PO or IV)
Hypermagnesemia	>2.5 mEq/L	CNS depression, hypoactive reflexes, flaccidity, respiratory depression, heart block, prolonged QT interval, hypotension, arrest	Identify high risk patients, ie, elderly or renal failure, calcium gluconate as antidote, increase fluids PO or IV, loop diuretic, hemodialysis

Cole, S. & Schaeffer, K. (Eds) (2008). *Portable fluids & electrolytes*. Philidelphia: Lippincott WIlliams & Wilkins.

Hemodynamic Algorithm

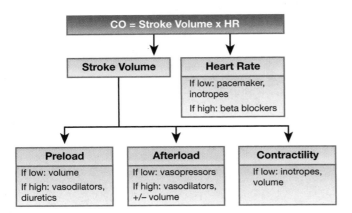

Mixed venous oxygen saturation normal 60–80%

Increases with: sepsis, alkalemia, hypometabolism

Decreases with: circulatory failure, cardiogenic shock, MI, pulmonary hypertension

Family Conference

Spikes 6-Step Protocol

Bring team together early, within the first week of admission to ICU. Consider having a premeeting with the team (physicians, nurses, dietician, physiotherapist, spiritual support, social worker, respiratory therapist) to ensure a consistent message using the same language is presented to the family.

Setting: ensure privacy, introduce team, allot adequate time

Perception: assess patient/family's understanding and expectations

Invitation: ask for permission from patient/family to share information

Knowledge: share knowledge about patient, clinical pathway; establish realistic goals

Emotion: respond to emotion with empathy

Summary: summarize information, establish follow-up plan, and document

---

Adapted from Treec, P. (2007). Communication in the intensive care unit about the end of life. *AACN Advanced Critical Care*, *18*(4), 406–414.